Aspen Culture
EDUCATION RESOURCES

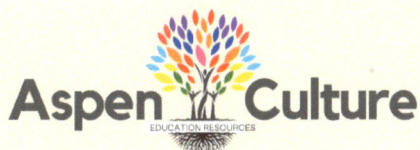

ASPEN CULTURE PUBLISHING

ISBN 978-0-578-304144

This Book Is Dedicated To My Family:

Together, we can move mountains!
Hooray to our first book! We did It!

#TeamSanders

# FROM OUR FAMILY TO YOURS:

Reading and learning together is one of the best ways to strengthen our connections at home. Our hope is that this book becomes a part of your daily affirmations to encourage and promote healthy habits for the physical and mental well being of the entire family.

A benefit index has been included in this book so that the reader can get a full understanding of the health benefits of each healthy choice.

More health! More life! More memories!

-Marleigh and Maria Sanders

i only have one body...

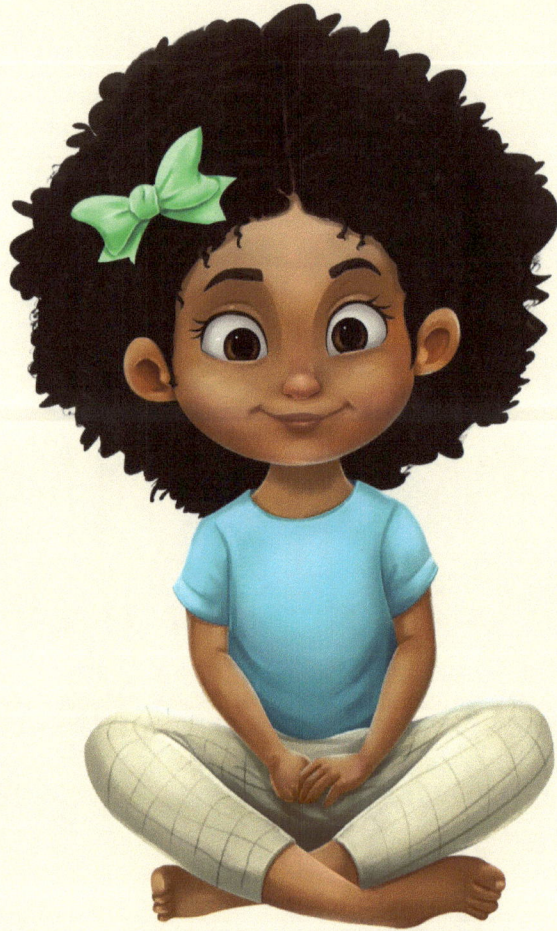

and it is up to me to LOVE my body.

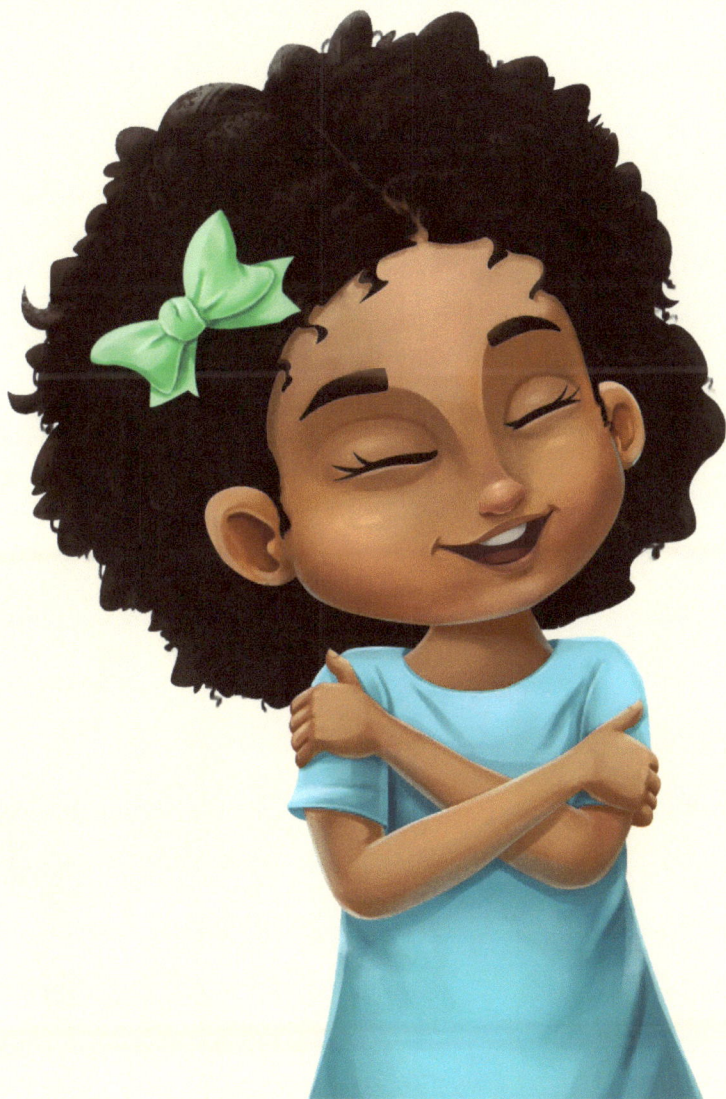

i love my body.

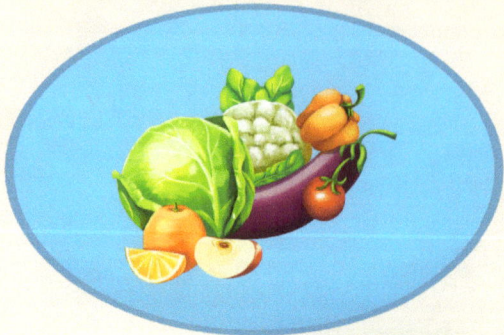

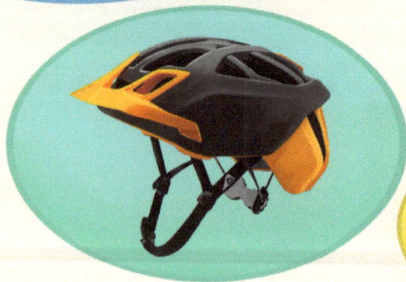

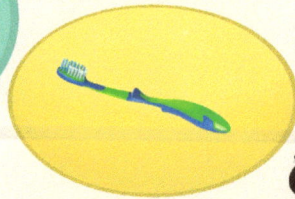

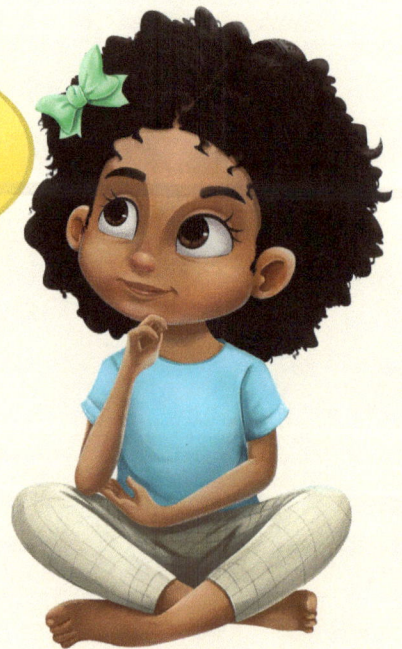

i make healthy choices for my body.

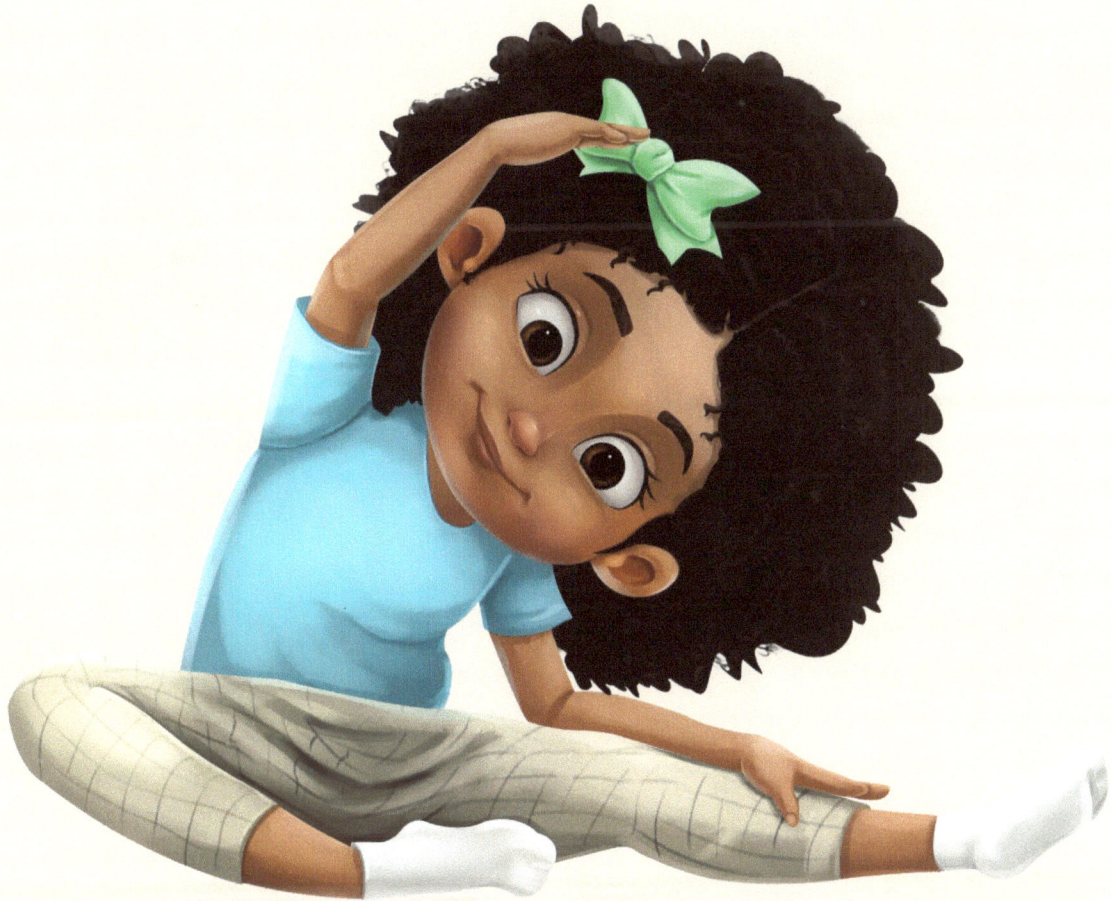

i stretch my body.

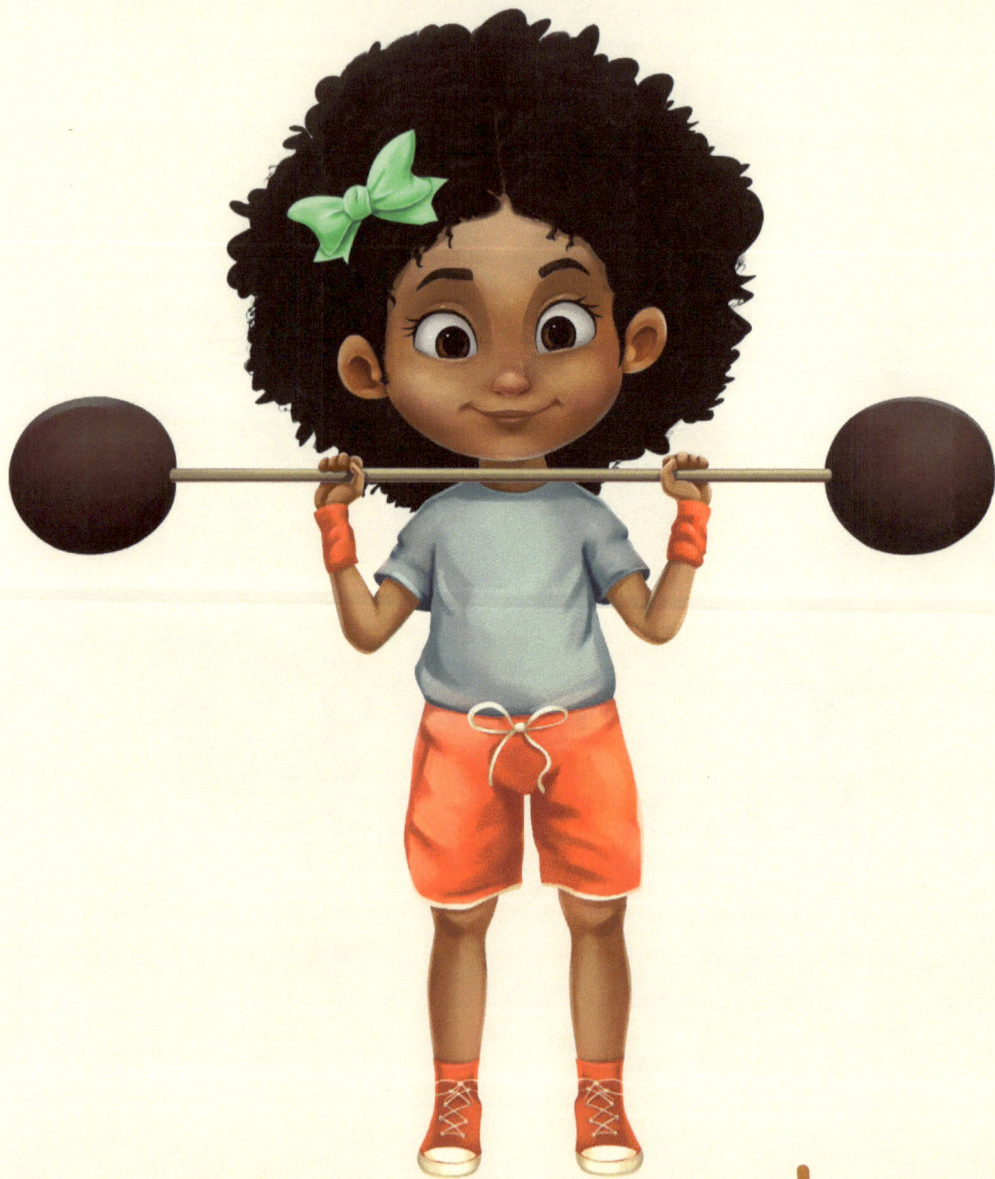

i exercise my body.

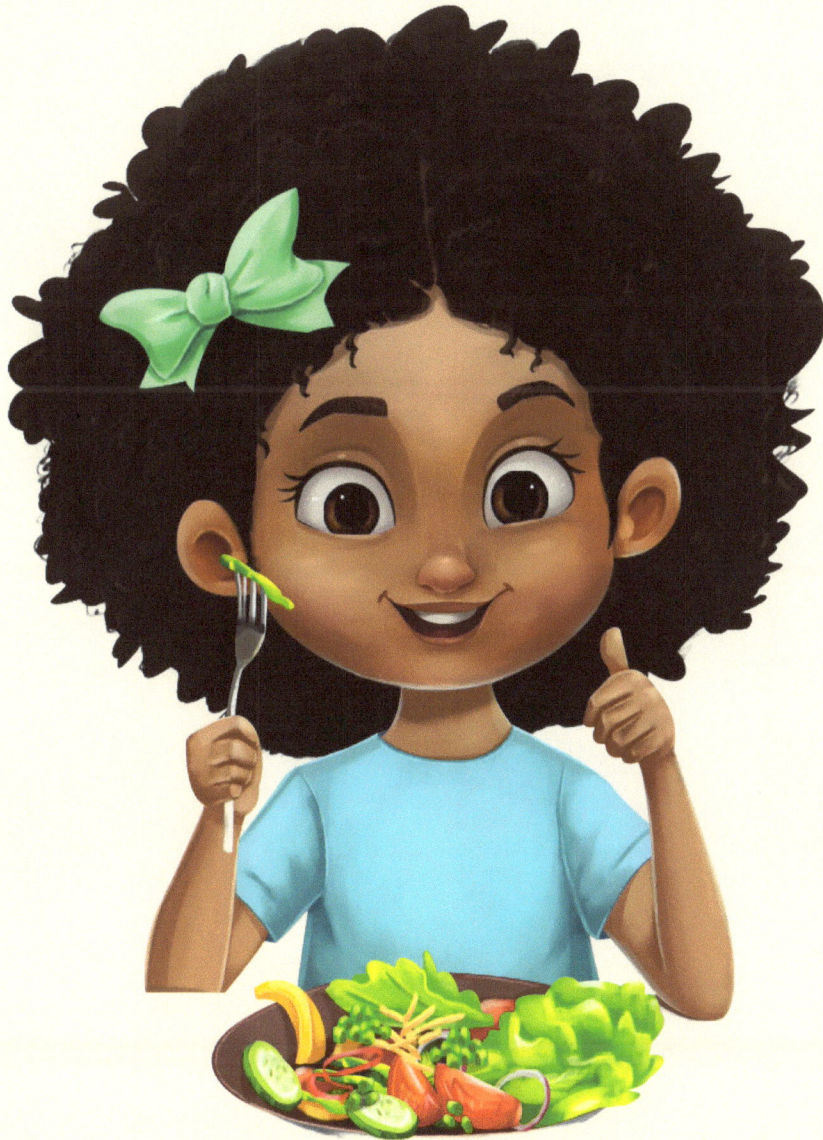

i eat veggies for my body.

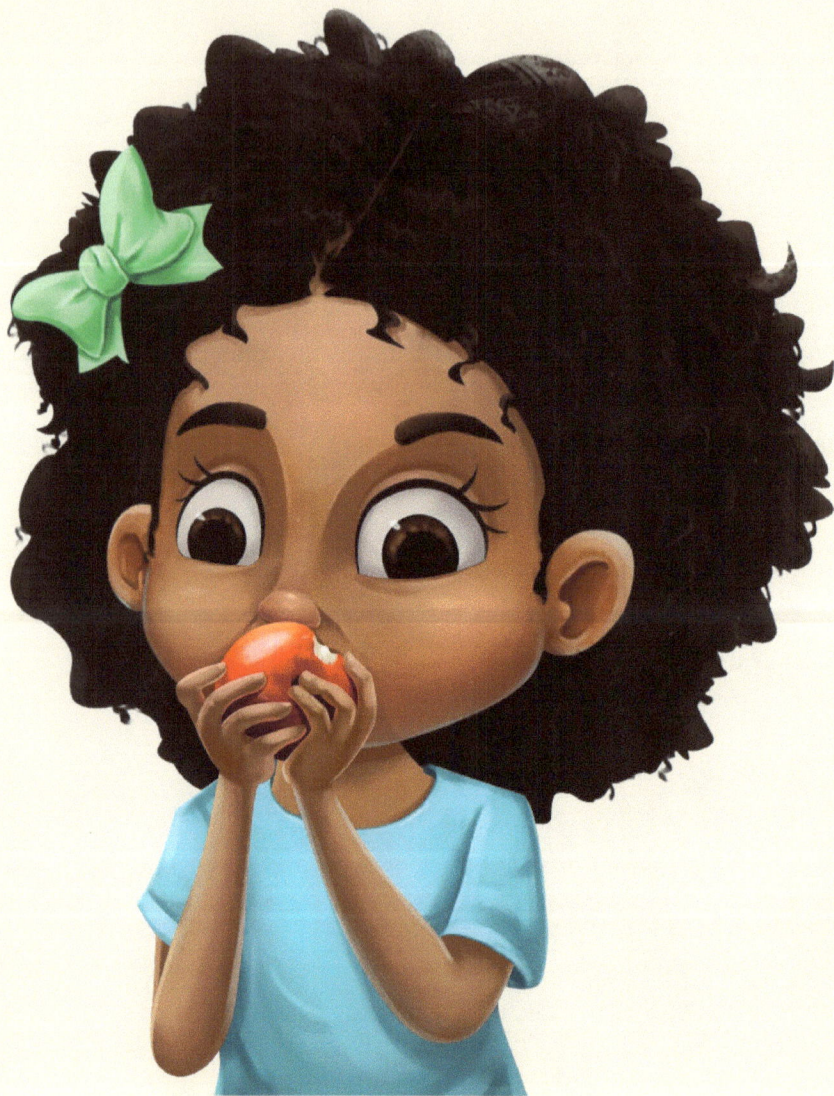

i eat fruits for my body.

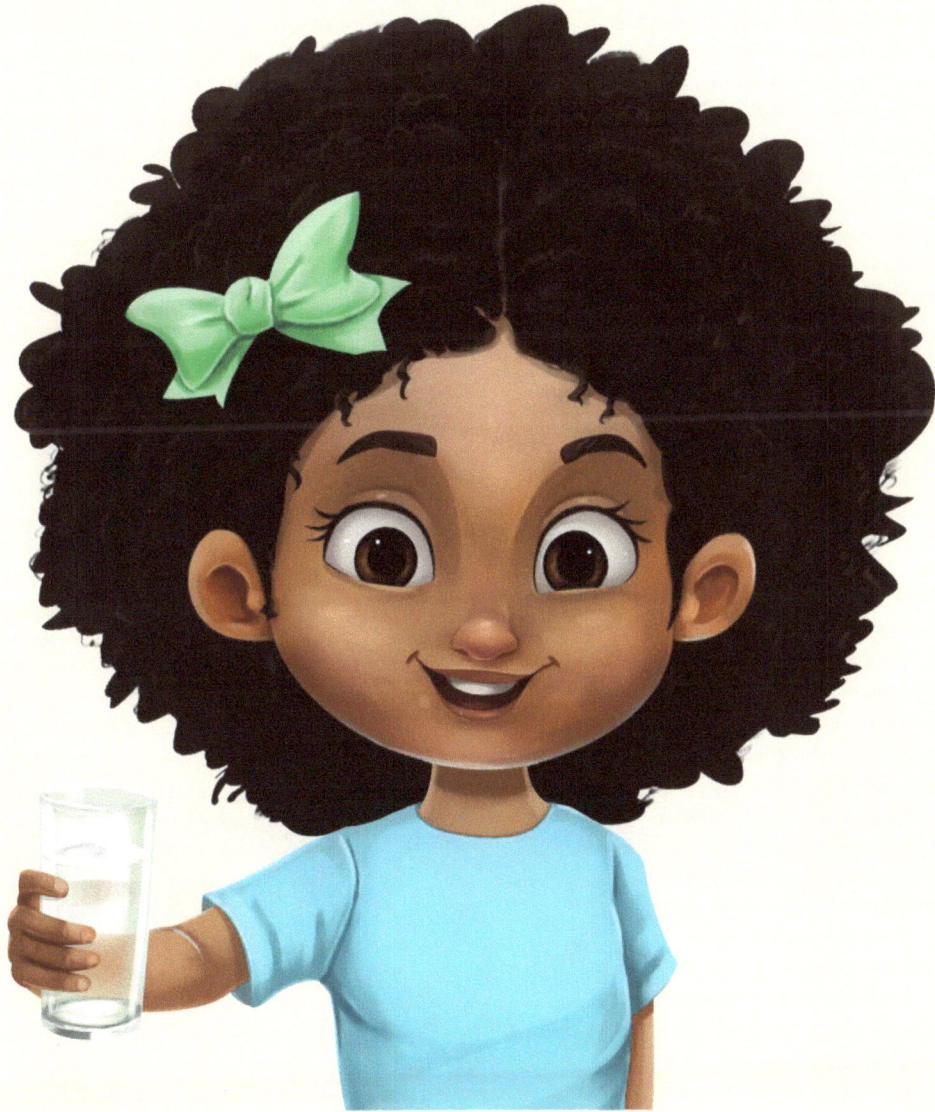

i drink water for my body everyday.

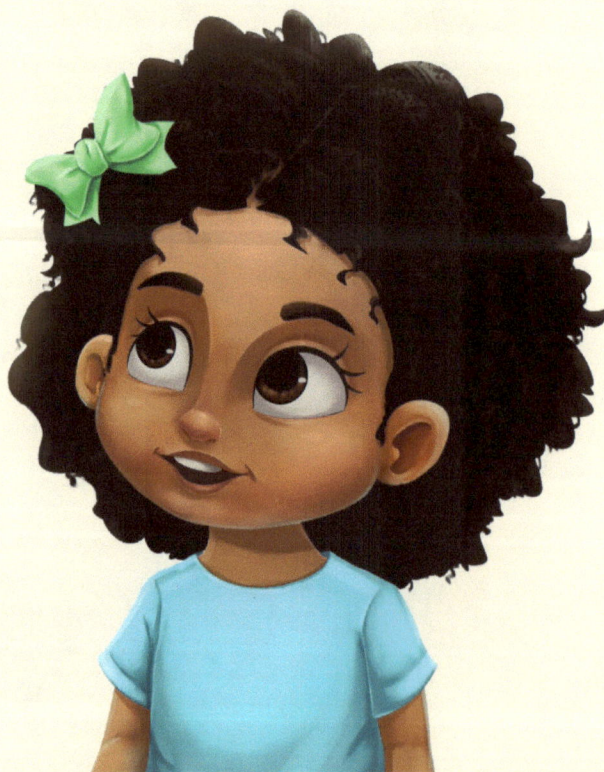

i give my body sunlight.

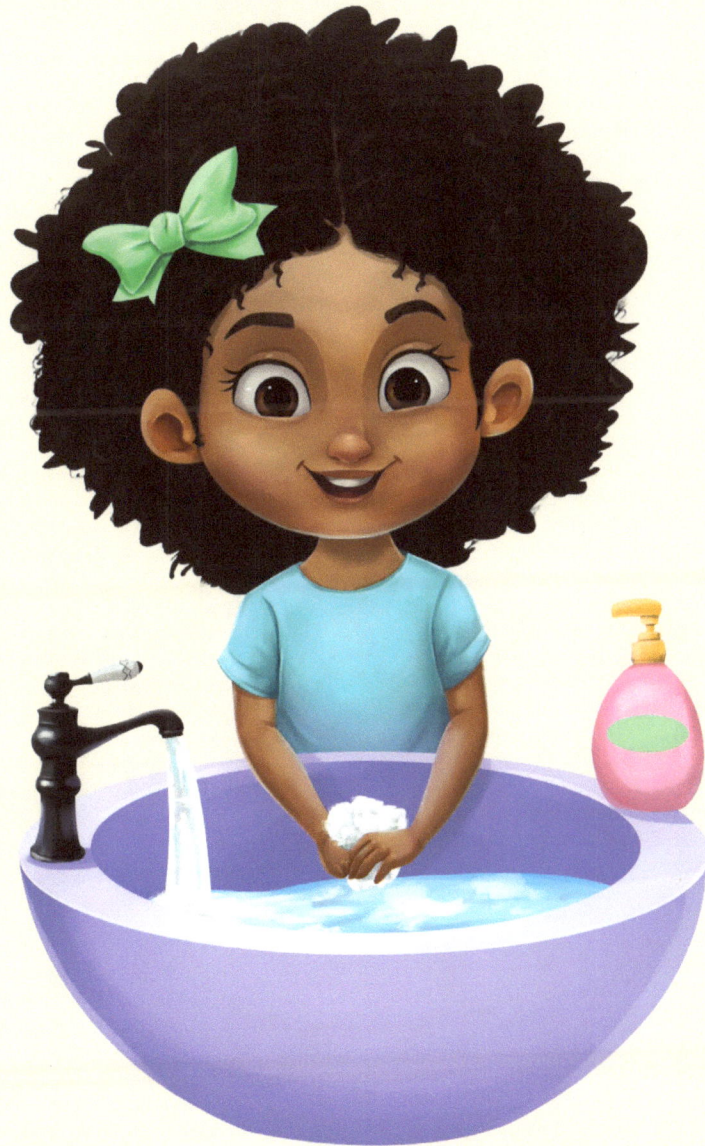

i clean my body.

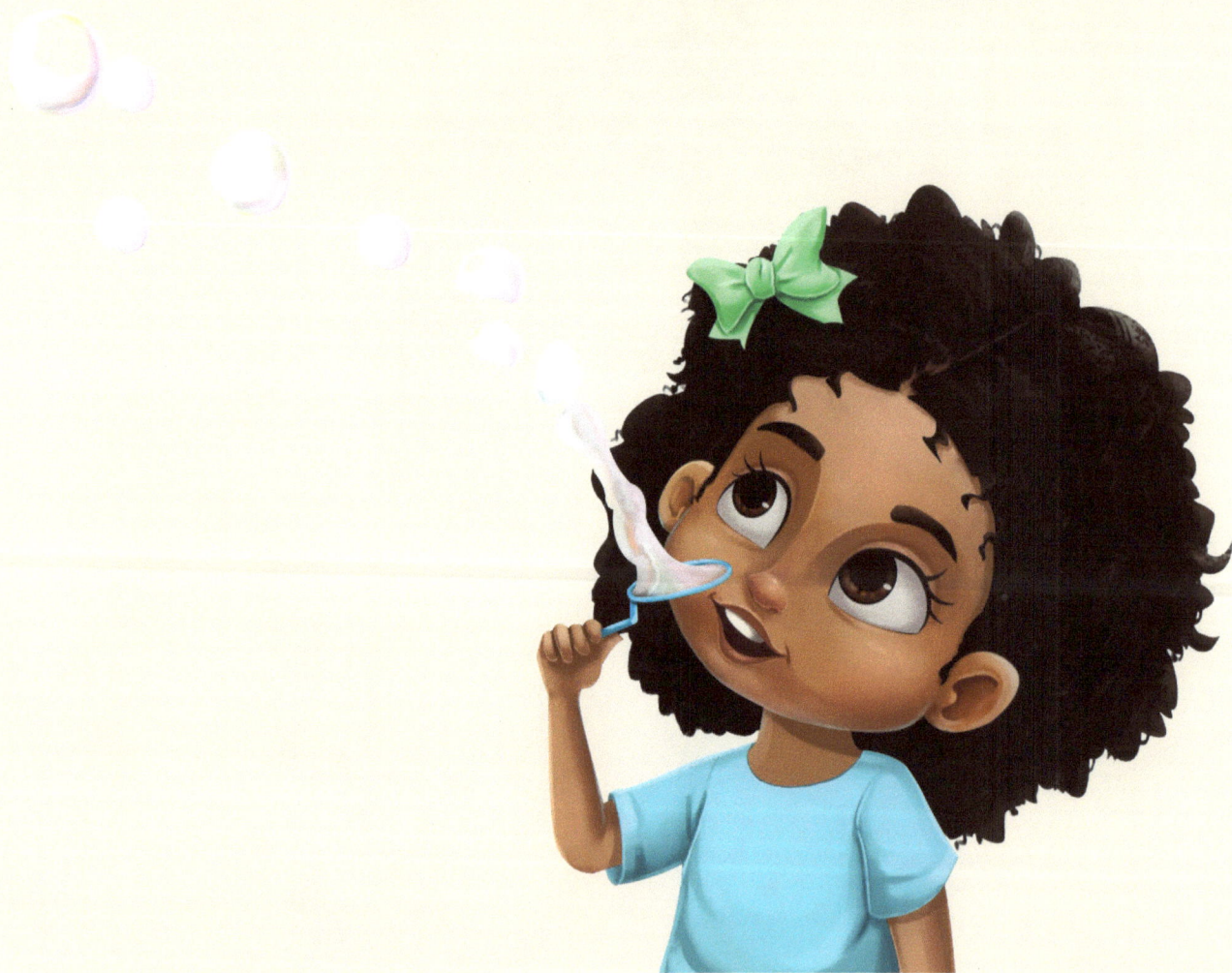

i am mindful of my body.

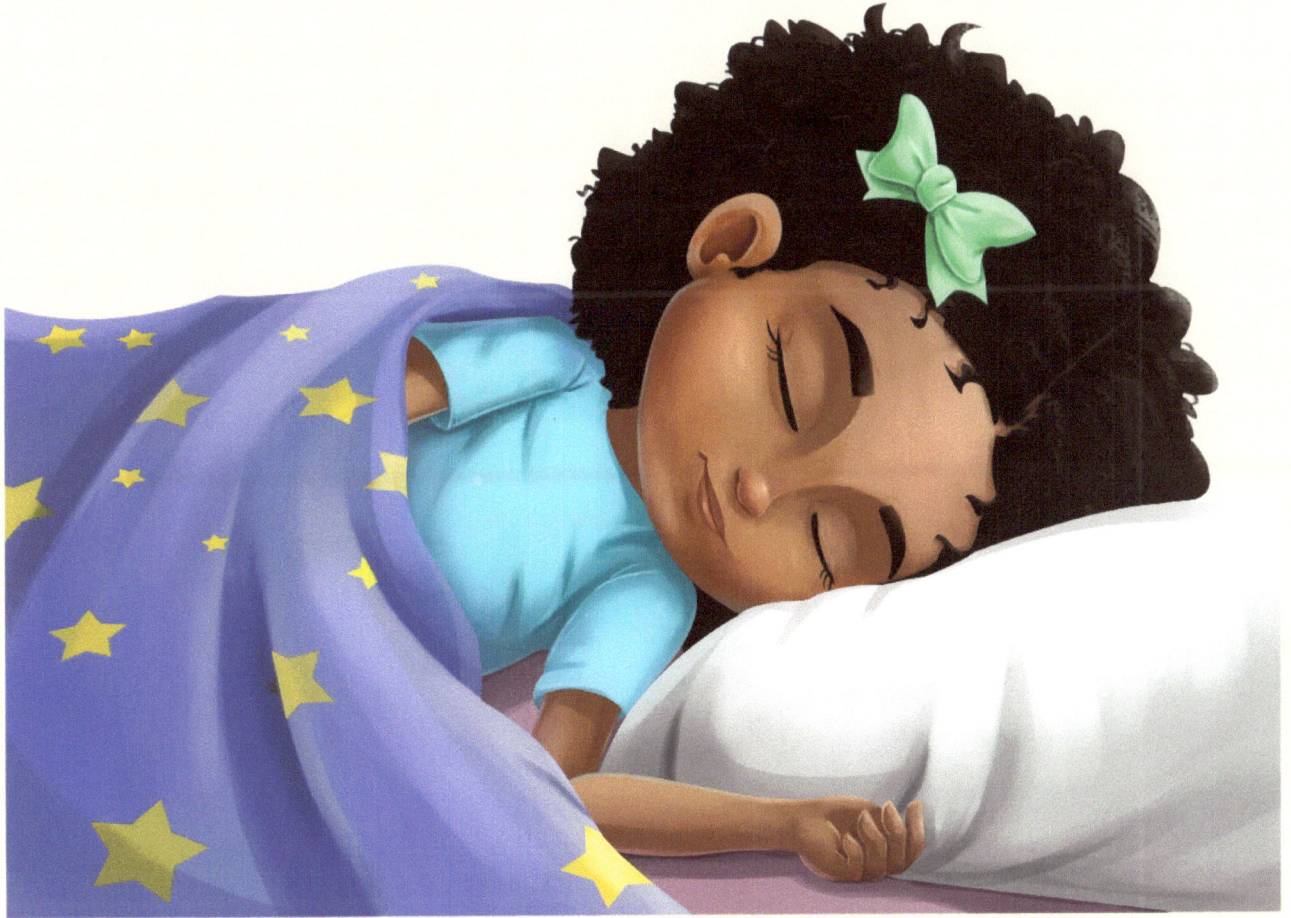

i rest my body.

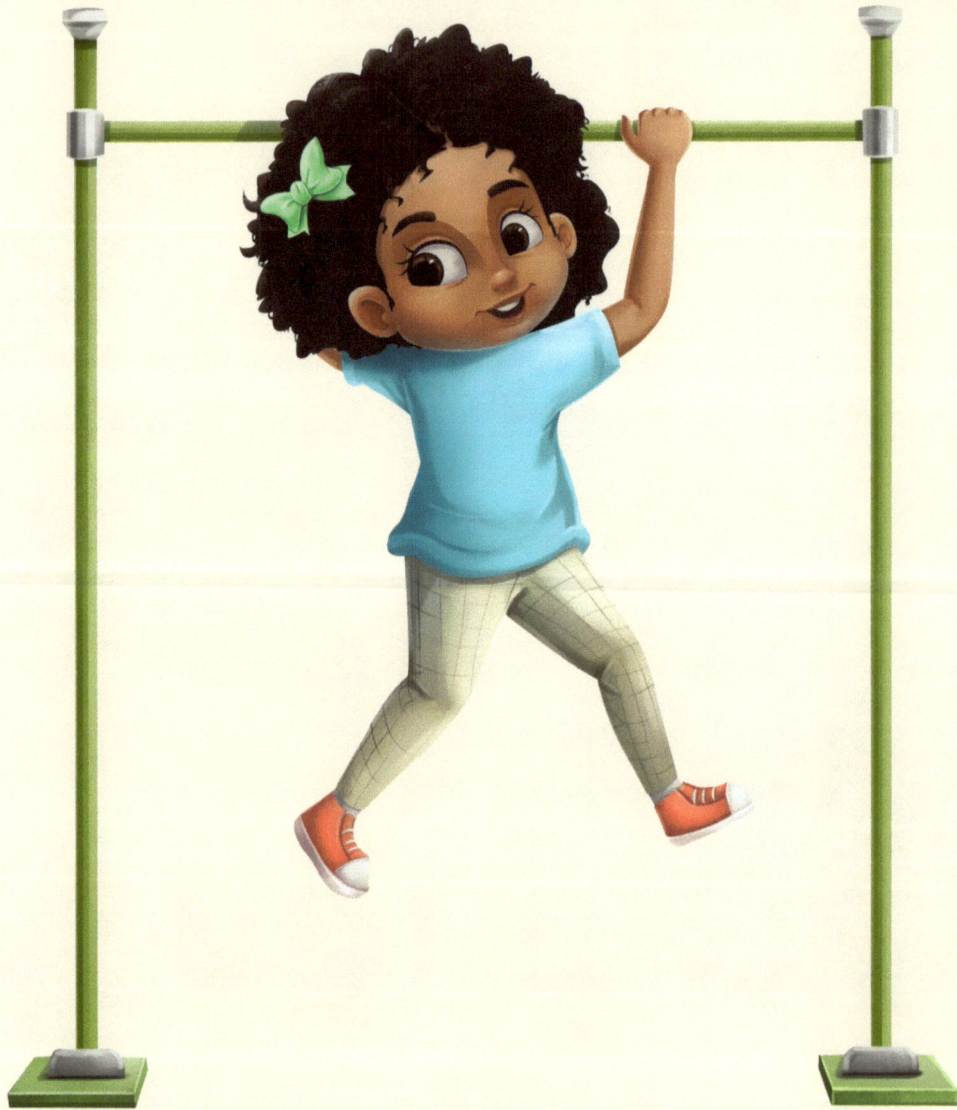

i challenge my body.

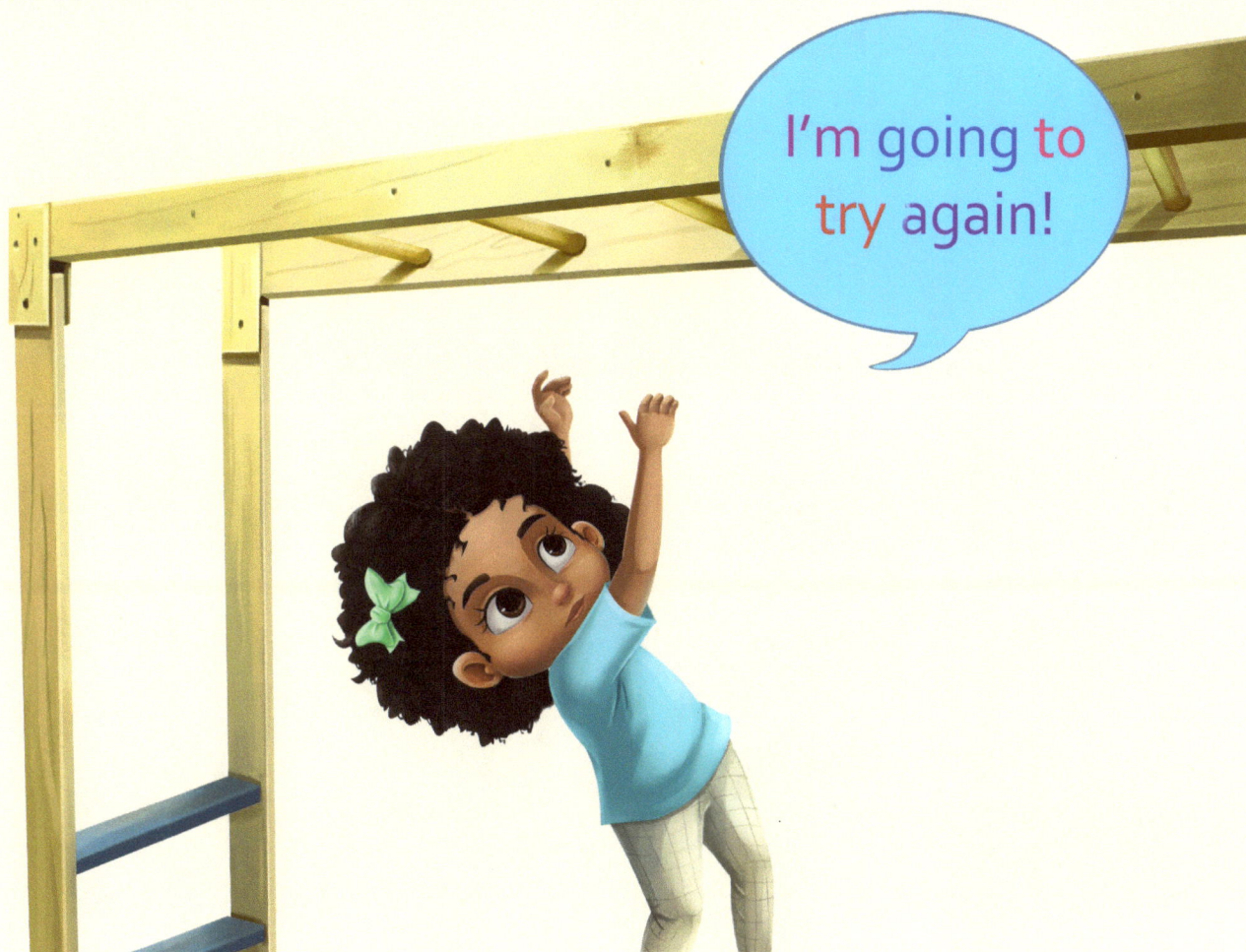

i am patient with my body.

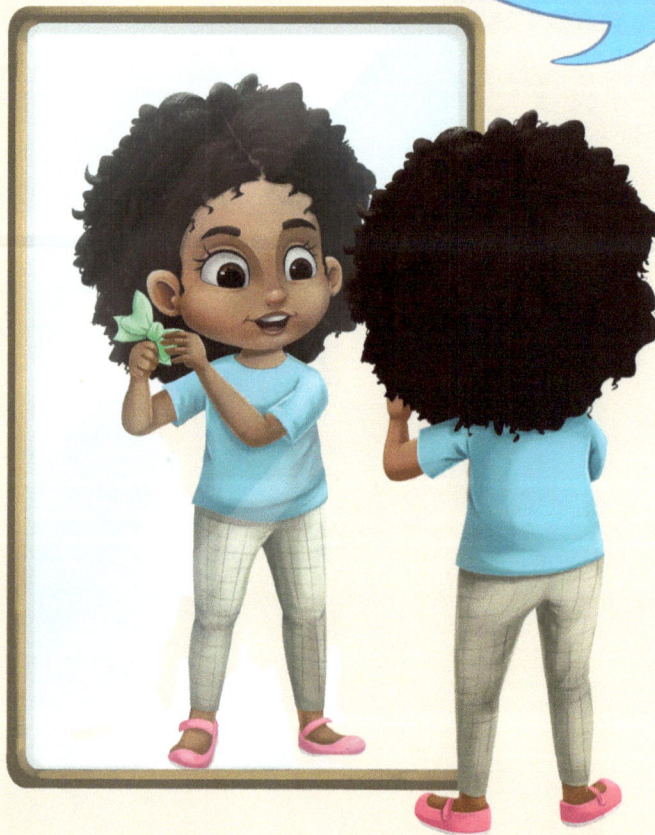

i say kind words to my body.

when i do these things...

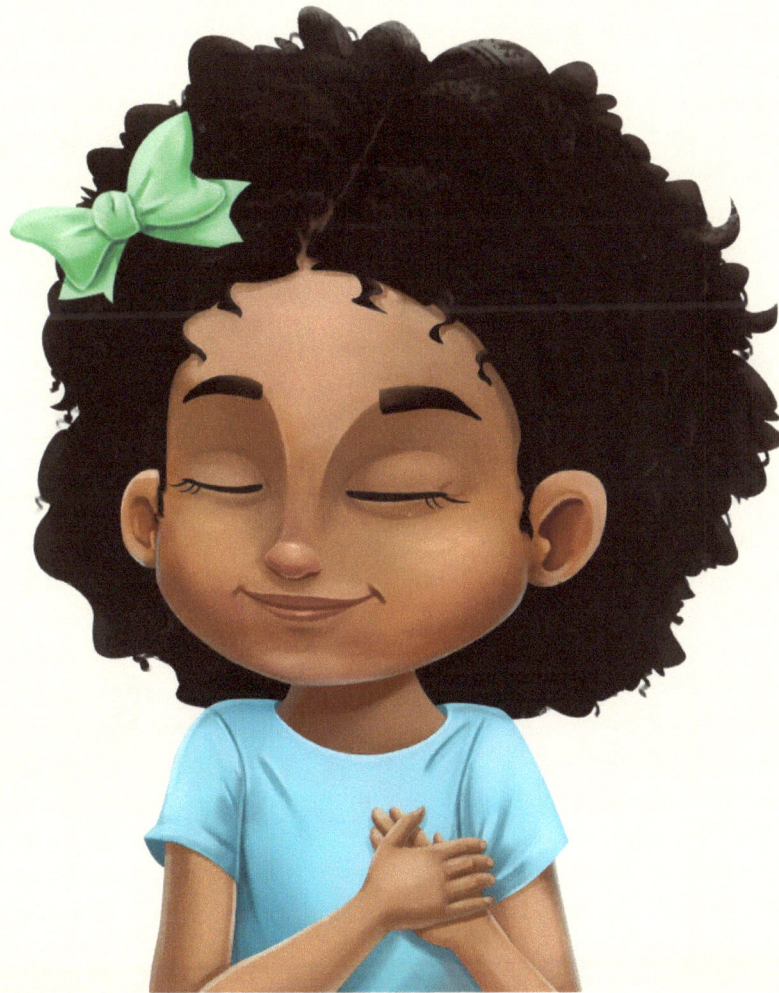

my body thanks me with strength, health, joy, and peace.

ONE BODY: A SELF-CARE
GUIDE FOR LITTLES

# benefit index

Learn about the benefits of each
healthy choice

# one body

## healthy choices

### benefits

- increases self-esteem
- increases productivity
- promotes positive attitude
- helps body to work at its fullest potential
- increases confidence
- increases decisiveness

## hygiene

### benefits

- increases self-esteem
- builds self-help skills
- prevents illnesses
- helps prevent the spread of germs
- helps prevent tooth decay
- improves overall health

## mindfulness

### benefits

- lowers stress and anxiety
- improves self-control
- improves attention and focus
- helps to develop resilience
- improves academic performance

# one body

## stretching

### benefits

- relieves stress
- lowers anxiety
- relieves sore muscles
- improves posture
- lowers risk of injury
- improves flexibility

## exercise

### benefits

- improves fitness
- increases concentration
- improves academic scores
- builds a stronger heart, bones and healthier muscles
- encourages healthy growth and development
- improves self-esteem
- improves posture and balance
- lowers stress
- improves sleep

## eating veggies

### benefits

- provides more energy
- boosts immunity
- keeps diabetes at bay
- keeps diseases at bay

# one body

## eating fruits

### benefits

- boosts immunity
- keeps obesity at bay
- keeps diseases away
- cleanses the body
- improves energy and performance

## drinking water

### benefits

- boosts metabolism
- prevents headaches
- promotes a healthy heart
- promotes healthy skin
- improves mood
- aids in weight loss
- increases energy
- improves digestion

## sunlight

### benefits

- improves mood
- boosts the immune system
- relieves pain
- promotes relaxation
- helps wounds heal
- helps people feel more alert
- supports better sleep
- reduces depression

# one body

## listening

### benefits

- promotes better decision making
- promotes self-knowledge
- helps you to learn your limits
- can save your life
- increases mindfulness
- improves relationship with your body

## rest

### benefits

- improves attention
- improves behavior
- improves learning
- improves memory
- improves mental health
- improves physical health

## challenge

### benefits

- promotes positive outlook on life
- trains the mind to be open to new ideas, new discoveries, and new opportunities
- improves self-esteem
- improves confidence
- builds resistance to the aging process

# one body

## being patient

### benefits

- increases productivity
- increases capacity for success
- make better decisions
- increases mindfulness
- better mental health
- improves relationships
- helps focus on long term goals

## kind words

### benefits

- reduces stress
- improves self-esteem
- increases motivation
- inspires productivity
- improves mental health
- improves physical health

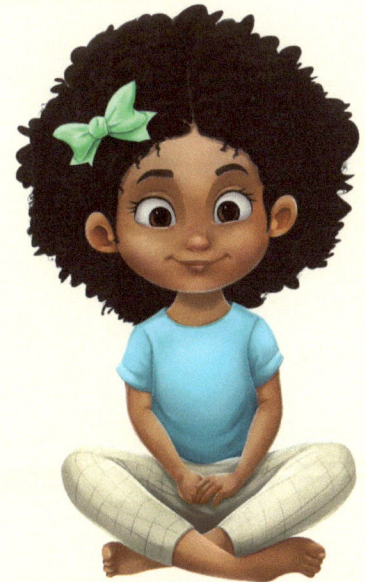

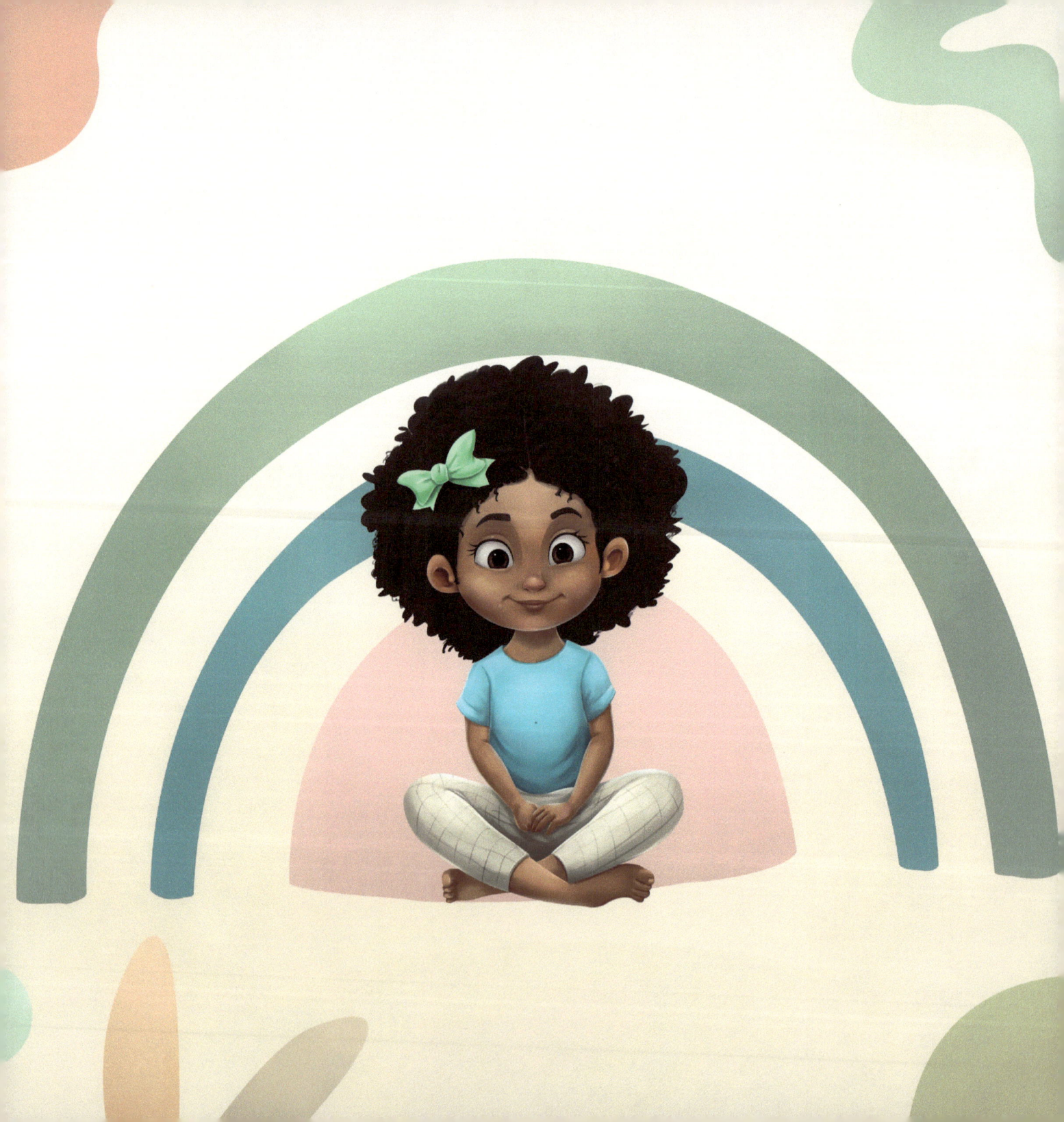